Life ——— with Anasofia

Anapaula Corral

Life—— with
Anasofia

Anapaula Corral

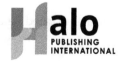

Halo
PUBLISHING
INTERNATIONAL

ISBN: 978-1-63765-147-6
LCCN: 2021922905

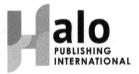

Halo Publishing International, LLC
www.halopublishing.com

In memory of my beloved
Abuelos Vico and Laura,
who were always my rock.

Contents

Preface

This book is neither a romantic tale nor a tragic story. Life with Anasofia is an account of an angel who graced this world only for a brief time but left a positive impact on the lives of those she touched.

She came to this world to remind us of how precious every second is – that we should cherish every moment before it fleets away, and when the moment came, she was gone. For the longest time, I wanted to write a book and pen down the words that can help someone suffering from loss, but every time I tried, I failed.

Most of the time, people fail to realize the necessary measures to take before conceiving a child. They are also unaware of the risks involved when you don't go to your routine appointments when sick. It is what motivated me to write this book.

Now, having penned down my feelings, hopefully my words can help bring you comfort in this world. In the book, I have written all my experiences and knowledge that I learned over time.

It can relate to you and your family experience or to some other trauma you may have suffered. I understand that nothing can cure the hurt you are going through, but trust that this, at least, can become an ointment to help heal your scar. Perhaps, it can help any family or friends that have experienced the same loss of a child or are going through the struggles of grief and loss of a loved one.

Chapter 1

The Parents Story

The Love Story of Her Mother and Father and Her Heritage

"You won't know what love is until you've loved deeply and lost deeply."

It is a common belief that once we find our one true love, we can get through anything in life. Mario and Isabel, thus, were lucky, for destiny itself had conspired to bring these soulmates together.

Although the love Mario and Isabel shared was different, the beginning of their story was like every other you may have read in the past. All the ingredients were present to make their existence vibrant and eventful. The life they cherished together was beautiful – not something we often see nowadays. From the moment they had laid eyes on each other, they knew their relationship would be unique.

They both were of twenty years when they first met each other. They were young, ambitious, their heads full of ideas, and their eyes sparkling with dreams. The foundation of their love set when they started working at the same place in Mexico City. They both were engaged in their lives and were devoted to building a career they could be proud of.

When they, Mario and Isabel, found each other, they were not looking for love. But for how long could they oppose their destiny?

Eventually, love lingered between them. The moment the two met, it did not take much time for them to become friends. From there, it was only a matter of time before their relationship graduated from being colleagues to partners. The connection was inevitable; their souls were the shards of the same being, and they yearned to be whole again. As love bloomed between them, they took no time to wait and embraced, requiting the feelings they had for each other. Their life had just started, yet with them now together, it already felt complete.

The moment they met, Mario and Isabel knew they were made for each other, and with that, they did not let anything come between them. It did not take long for either of them to realize they wanted to be with each other every step of the way. And so, naturally, they decided to get married.

With a deep and profound love having emerged between them, they wanted to commemorate that love, to make their relationship endless. They knew it was time for them to get married and, with Cupid's blessing, sign the pact that will bind ever closer.

On the day of their wedding, they knew they would always be together. Life was good to them, and they were both loyal to each other. The prospect of life forever with one another felt exciting and rapturous. They were delighted. They had multiple plans and dreams they wanted to achieve together, and for that, they also planned to leave Mexico City. They loved God, and they knew that the bond they shared was inseparable.

The joy of being young and the possibility of a promising future was unmistakably there. They did not think twice that the decision to get married was the one they would ever look back at with regret.

Now, let me warn you: this is not a love story and neither an emotional one.

All of us want endless love. We have notions of affection; one is our optimal notion while the other is the real notion. Mario and Isabel cooperated to make their love perpetual. For them, love meant being in the company of each other. However, once the two got married and started to live together, their relationship began to change. It did not take a turn for the worse, but they began to understand just how much destiny affected the lives they led. For them, this relationship was all thanks to "The fate of love."

On this strange, yet terrifically substantial subject, there was a highlighted center; it was the reality of their karmic relationship. Mario and Isabel were encountering another sort of affection, one they had never felt. Their bond nearly felt like an attractive association; it was drawing them into one another. Like two magnets, it pulled them closer. In any case, their relationship was not merely cherished.

At the start, it was filled with passion and emotions, but then, one day, there came pain. This balance between pain and passion often happened at the same time. For them, love did not come without its many effects. It was a result of so many things, so many emotions. Most importantly, the love these two found was a result of their past actions and different upbringings. They both had family differences as well that ultimately influenced the love they felt in their lives.

It was not just limited to romance; it was in everything. In a relationship, karma refers to this life and the droplets of so many other lifetimes. If you are a believer of the age-old saying, "what goes around comes around," just like the two of them, you are also a believer in destiny. Every word of this concept was of importance.

They tried to understand everything about their relationship. However, that is not how love works. Love is rarely ever understood. To better understand how fate influenced Mario and Isabel and the importance of love in their lives, it is helpful to look at it as a higher concept.

For Mario, Isabel was someone who he craved to be with. Even after being together for years, he could never understand what brought them together. If they did not suffer the loss they were going to face in the future, he would think their pure, endless love resulted from all the good deeds in their past lives. However, this was not the case. Mario and Isabel's love was not filled with only high points.

If you have always been a good person, it doesn't guarantee a seamless love life. No matter who you are or what you have done, love remains a tricky business. If only one starts to count all the present concepts (a nod to Shakespeare), this whole love thing can get so messed up, entangled, and yet, be so sweet. Every human being, regardless of who they are, has a beginning, a middle, and an end. Similarly, every relationship has a similar setting. Karmic relationships essentially are stretched out in a way that people, who come across them, learn something from them.

Moreover, even if you and your significant other are meant to be like Mario and Isabel, your relationship can still take a dip into the water of the karmic sphere. They soon realized that not everything about their relationship was built on love and attraction. Like any other marriages, they discerned theirs had flaws as well. Maybe these few flaws were not a bad thing. Perhaps the process of working together and building this relationship was vetting them for what the future held before Anasofia came to this world. Nothing in life can be flawless, especially relationships. It is a constant work in progress, but they were both willing to put in the work for "The One."

Sure, they had their ups and downs. There were parts of it that had their cracks. There were days the two did not like each other, but there was never a day they did not love each other. No matter what obstacle stood in front of them, it never seemed big enough to dull the spark between the two. It takes a second to break a relationship, but it takes years of hard work, dedication, and sacrifice to make it work. This is what Mario and Isabel believed in. They trusted God, they trusted destiny, and most importantly, they trusted each other. It was the ideal recipe for happiness.

The bond they shared was innate, natural, universal, and eternal. Days, months, and years passed in their relationship, yet no matter the obstacle, the love between them never changed. Not once did they have feelings of wanting to leave each other. If it was possible, it was now somewhat more assertive.

Their story was with its faults, too, but it was never significant enough to cause any significant problems. Their guts told them things would be hard; it is often said that something peculiar waited for them in the future. But the love between the two was enough in more ways than one. Their passion soon became exemplary. It gave the people who knew them a sense that they were in the presence of love. When Mario and Isabel were together, their need for love was more significant than ever. The kind of love they shared was an example for all those around them. It was stimulating, and it was easy for their friends and family to feel happy for them.

Their love journey might look complete to some, but it did not begin with Mario and Isabel. It started with Anasofia!

Their relationship was a vessel for Anasofia, and they gave her all the love they could as soon as she was born. They wanted to share the abundance that they had with another entity that was now blooming in the comfort of their hearts. Her parents loved her in every way they could; they knew she was a special child. They could sense her prominence.

She came into their lives like a thread that connected the two of them and made them stronger. Because of her presence, the love between the two grew exponentially.

Anasofia's life became meaningful because she could sense how loving her parents were. Their passion was whole, the kind that is read about only in books. With each passing day, it kept growing. Anasofia was a gift sent to them from God to enrich their lives.

The foundation of their love and marriage was built on reciprocity and commitment. The union of their beings was based uniquely on love and respect.

Anasofia blessed their lives with more meaning than they knew possible. Her essence bound them together in a way no other experience could. She completed their already wholesome lives. These incredible feelings of intimacy held them together, and they showed to the world through their love in the form of Anasofia. Moreover, they committed to making each other feel loved and comfortable.

They knew it was love because even when faced with uncomfortable situations in their life, they held to each other. Despite the obstacles, they wanted to be together with each other every step of the way. You know you love someone when you focus on each other's needs, and they did. They were not selfish, and they had genuinely fallen in love with each other.

Living is hard, but the love we share with those who likewise adore and care about us makes our life experiences so much better.

It is not always an easy task to love someone and share your life with them, nor is it continually benevolent. Still, it is the most beautiful feeling in the world. Knowing the relationship that the two of them shared was one of the most inspiring things to witness for everyone around them.

Chapter 2

The Sparkle of Life

How She Was Conceived

It was not long after her honeymoon when Isabel noticed hormonal changes in her body, and from that moment, she knew she was carrying a life inside of her. Mothers will always get that special feeling when they realize they are expecting a baby. In Isabel's case, she knew it was more than that – it was something different.

Before we get into the story, I will ask you a few questions you may not have pondered. Have any of your relatives had health problems that tend to run in families? What do you know about your family tree? Which of these problems affected your parents or grandparents? Which health conditions might you pass on to your children? Thanks to advances in medical research, doctors now have the tools to understand how certain illnesses, or increased risks illnesses, pass from generation to generation.

Instead of being appreciative, most of us take good health for granted when we talk about health. It is also essential to understand that our bodies contain a unique set of chemical blueprints that affect their looks and functions. These chemical blueprints are present in our DNA (deoxyribonucleic acid). It's round-elongated molecules containing nucleotides – linked pieces – carry the codes for genetic information.

I know I may have gotten a bit more technical there, but do not worry. Let me simplify it for you. Whenever a woman is pregnant with a baby girl – like Isabel, her DNA will already be present in the child because everyone's DNA carries a genetic code that passes from generation to generation.

Genes are perfectly bundled inside the structures, alongside the portions of our DNA called chromosomes. Each human cell contains 46 chromosomes, orchestrated as 23 sets (called autosomes). After conceiving (when a sperm cell and an egg meet up to make an infant), the chromosomes repeatedly copy to give similar hereditary data to each new cell in creating the life. Twenty-two autosomes are the equivalent of males and females. Likewise, females have two X chromosomes, and males have one X and one Y chromosome. The X and the Y are known as sex chromosomes. Human chromosomes are sufficiently huge to be seen with a powerful magnifying instrument, and the 23 sets can be distinguished by differences in their size, shape, and manner.

Sometimes even when you are perfectly healthy, problems can arise. The human body is complex, and this process of Child Birth that we all take for granted can go wrong. I hope and pray that no mother has to go through these problems ever. However, many do. Many mothers can have problems because of errors in the genetic code or "gene recipe." These errors sometimes don't look like anything crucial to a mind that does not understand it, but they can happen in a variety of ways.

Your genetic code consists of a lot of pieces of information. Information that is vital and that makes a person. Sometimes when that genetic code is being written down, some vital information can go missing from the code. However, there is also the possibility of this genetic code having an overburden of information or having information that's in the wrong order. These errors can be devastating.

Let us take a look at an example that might make it easier to understand. Pretend there is a recipe that you are trying to make for the first time, but when you note down the recipe, you miss a few ingredients. Now the entire recipe has changed. We need to understand that behind the scenes, things are happening that can change the setup of our bodies. So, regardless of whether these errors in your genetic makeup ate big or small, the outcome can be noteworthy, and these concerns can cause a person to have a disability or at risk of a shortened life span.

When a mistake occurs in the genetic information while a cell is dividing, it can cause further problems. Sometimes it can error in the number of chromosomes a person has. The developing embryo then grows and gets life from cells that either have too many chromosomes or not enough.

Now, really put your mind to the test and think about it. Every time we think about the process of pregnancy, the changes one's body goes through, the complications a mother faces, we never really know about all these intricate details of childbirth that are going on inside the mother as she's creating this life. We never think about how detail-oriented this whole process is. There are hundreds of things that can go wrong, yet more often than not, they don't. But for that one couple that does go through these complications, it gets harder to ignore these details.

Normally when it comes to chromosomes, each parent gives 23 chromosomes. When the sperm of a man fertilizes an egg inside of a woman, the union leads to a baby with 46 chromosomes. This is when normal meiosis takes place. However, what we do not think about is that things can go wrong, even at this initial stage. In trisomy, there are three copies of a couple's chromosome. The body multiplies one particular chromosome three times instead of the standard two.

There is Trisomy 21, which is known as Down syndrome. There is Trisomy 18 called Edwards syndrome, and also Trisomy 13 known as Patau syndrome. These are all examples of this genetic problem that might happen when there is a mix-up in chromosomes.

Edwards syndrome is a genetic disorder, and it affects one out of every 7,500 births. Babies born with this syndrome have a low birth weight and small head, mouth, jaw, and heart defects. The hands of a baby suffering from Edwards Syndrome typically form clenched fists, and their fingers overlap each other instinctively. Unfortunately, new research shows that they might also have other birth defects involving the hips and feet, heart, kidney problems, and intellectual disability that restricts their mental growth.

This disorder is heartbreaking. When you give birth to a child that has a third copy of chromosome 18, the chances of that baby surviving decrease dramatically. Only about 5% of children suffering from Edwards Syndrome live long enough to celebrate their first birthday.

Then there is Trisomy 13, unlike Trisomy 18, when a baby has an extra 13th chromosome. This genetic complication affects couples a lot less than Trisomy 18. This can affect one out of every 15,000 to 25,000 births. Children with this condition also suffer from physical disabilities. They often have cleft lip and palate, which is usually a V-shaped indented formation. They can have other foot abnormalities, like an extra toe, and many different structural abnormalities of the skull and face. Apart from physical disabilities, this condition also causes birth defects of the ribs, heart, abdominal organs, and sex organs. Long-term survival is unlikely but possible.

In **monosomy**, unlike trisomy, there isn't anything extra. In fact, in this form of numerical error, one member of a chromosome pair is missing hence the word 'mono.' To put it simply, there are fewer chromosomes, rather than too many.

A baby with a missing autosome has a very small chance of survival. However, if a baby is missing a sex chromosome, then the baby can survive in certain cases. One example is Turner syndrome, a condition that only affects girls. It is when girls are born with just one X chromosome. They might face development and a few physical challenges like short height and failure of the ovaries. With proper medication and care, these girls can live productive lives as long as they seek medical care for any health problems that arise with their condition.

However, sometimes, other problems can arise too. When the number of chromosomes is not the problem, the chromosomes themselves can have something wrong, like an added or missing part. When a part of the information is missing from a chromosome, it's called a deletion. Deletion is visible on a chromosome under a microscope. When it is too tiny to be visible, it is called a microdeletion.

In almost four hundred newborns, there are bits and pieces of chromosomes that shift from one to another in areas of the chromosome called translocations. When information from one chromosome goes to another, it confuses the entire system. While most translocations are categorized as "balanced," meaning there is neither gain nor loss of genetic material, unfortunately, not every newborn baby is that lucky. Because in some, there are "unbalanced" chromosomes, which means there may be too much genetic material in some places while there is not enough in others.

When a problem occurs in the genetic makeup of a child, small parts of the DNA code can seem to be taken out almost with the snip of a scissor. In one out of every 100 newborns, these inversions or reversals are flipped over and reinserted. These chromosome abnormalities of translocations can either be inherited from a parent but sometimes happens spontaneously in a child's own chromosomes regardless of the child's parents.

The good thing is deletions do not cause any physical disabilities. Both balanced translocations and inversions, according to many pieces of research, cause no abnormalities of shape, form, or developmental problems in the kids who suffer from either of the two.

However, those with deletions, whether it is translocations or inversions, might have a few complications later on in life. That means any individual born with deletion who chooses to become a parent later on in life may have an increased risk of miscarriage or chromosome abnormalities in their children.

Then there is another subject that most parents know absolutely nothing out. In a lot of cultures, sex is one thing that's not in a person's hands. And, to a certain extent, that statement is true, but our bodies contribute to the gender of the child. And, these chromosomes that certify a child's sex can also be responsible for causing problems. In simple terms, these genetic problems in children can come to the surface when abnormalities affect the sex chromosomes.

Usually, a child will be a male when he inherits one X chromosome from his mother and one Y chromosome from his father. On the other hand, a child will be a female if she inherits two X's (one from each parent) and zero Y chromosomes.

Sometimes, there may be an instance when children are born with only one sex chromosome. Typically that one chromosome is X, but sometimes a child can be born with an extra X or Y.

Girls with Turner syndrome that we talked about before are an example of children with one chromosome. In contrast, boys suffering from Klinefelter syndrome are born with one or more extra X chromosomes (XXY or XXXY).

Sometimes, a genetic problem is X-linked, meaning that this abnormality was because of the X chromosome. This type of abnormality in children is known as Fragile X syndrome, a genetic disorder that causes intellectual disability in boys. Then other diseases can be carried by or on the X chromosome, including hemophilia and Duchenne muscular dystrophy. All three of these abnormalities primarily affect boys.

It's not to say that this abnormality of the X chromosome can happen to girls. It can, and Females can also be carriers of these diseases. However, the only difference is since they also inherit one normal X chromosome, the gene change effects are minimal. However, males only have one X-chromosome and are almost always the ones who show the X-linked disorder's full impact.

Babies can also suffer because of another thing called gene mutation. Some problems are caused by a single gene that is present but is altered in some way. To understand it better, think of it like a book you get. However, all the other books with the same title have the same writing in them, but yours does not. Even though the writing is present, it is altered in some way. Such changes in genes are called mutations or gene variants.

Any time there is a mutation in a gene, the chromosomes' number and appearance are usually still standard. And, just like the problems caused by other chromosomes, a genetic mutation in your child is also not good news. Many genetic illnesses can be caused by one problem gene. These diseases include phenylketonuria (PKU), cystic fibrosis, sickle cell disease, Tay-Sachs disease, and achondroplasia (a type of dwarfism).

Although experts used to think that errors in a single gene caused no more than 3% of all human diseases, new research shows that this is underestimated. Within the last few years, scientists have discovered genetic links to many different conditions that weren't originally thought of as genetic, including Parkinson's disease, Alzheimer's disease, heart disease, diabetes, and several different types of cancer. Alterations in these genes are thought to increase one's risk of developing these conditions; however, studying these genes has led to a better understanding of the human body.

Then there is another gene which is known as the cancer-causing-gene. After researching genetic mutation, doctors have identified 50 cancer-causing genes that significantly increase a person's odds of developing cancer. Using sophisticated tests, doctors can identify who has these cancer-causing genetic mutations, and determine who is at risk, potentially saving their life. For example, scientists have concluded that colorectal cancer (cancer that occurs in the colon or rectum) is sometimes associated with mutations in a gene called APC. Along with this, they have also discovered that abnormalities in the BRCA1 and BRCA2 genes increase the risk of developing breast cancer and increase the risk for ovarian tumors by 50%.

However, with changes in technology, doctors can carefully monitor people known to have these gene mutations now. If problems develop over time, people with this genetic makeup are more likely to get treated for cancer a lot earlier. This early diagnosis has enabled doctors to provide better care to their patients and increase the quality of life for those suffering from these genetic conditions.

When Anasofia was conceived she had an extra love chromosome which contributed to her physical being but not her spiritual one. Mario and Isabel were well aware of this since the day she was born. She was special and they all knew it. If today you have or know someone that has a child with an extra chromosome, I encourage you to keep on reading.

Chapter 3

Her Name, Her legacy

Her Soul Mission

Names, not a lot of people think about them, but they're one of the most important parts of you. Think about it; someone's name is how you know them; it is how you call them. Every name tells a story of who we are, what we shall be and become. Therefore, as parents, when naming our children, we should think very carefully about it as the name will go on to deeply impact our children as they grow up.

You are your name.

If today you do not know the meaning or origin of your name, I strongly suggest you do find out. It will make you know yourself in a way nothing else has. It might sound outdated, but your name has a significant impact on your personality. It is not just a popular belief, but it makes sense that names that are negative and have negative connotations will not inspire a child to develop positively or have a good outcome in life. The child will not grow to make a positive contribution to their community.

Therefore, as parents, let us not wait for our children to cry out to God or face adversity in life before we act. You have every means available to you to search for the best name possible, to search for a name that describes your bond, that will identify this beautiful soul you and your loved one have created.

As parents, we must ensure that we give our children the best we can afford emotionally, mentally, education- ally, physically, and financially to install positivity in them. So that they can be proud of us as parents and become hon- orable citizens in our community. So why not start with choosing a name that will bring them eternal happiness and prominence?

My plea to all parents is this. Be wise and choose for your children good, honorable, and positive names. When it was Mario's and Isabel's time to choose a name, they wanted it to be special. The moment they knew they were expecting a baby girl, they wanted to name her something that displayed how they truly felt, how they wanted to embody this child of theirs.

They searched everywhere to know what the name meant. They must have looked through hundreds if not thousands of names to find one that just felt like theirs. After so many days of spiraling and searching, Isabel and Mario came to name their precious child Anasofia. The name Ana is of Spanish origin, meaning Gracious or Merciful, and this is why they named her that because they were grateful to have their little Ana.

Ana is a name used primarily by parents considering baby names for girls that have a higher meaning – ones that are more than just a sound. It is a name that has been used for centuries. Sometimes, through the years, it was spelled differently. Old Testament translations, including English ones, use *Hannah* or sometimes *Channah* instead of Anna. However, they mean the same thing.

When they inquired further, everything about the first name appealed to them. It had a religious feeling, as the name appears for a short time in the New Testament. This time, the name belonged to a prophetess who recognized Jesus as the Messiah.

That's not all. Anna was a popular name after that as well. In the Byzantine Empire from an early date in the Middle Ages, Anna became a status symbol. It was a name used to differentiate between people and their religious values. Slowly as the years progressed, the name became common among Western Christians due to the veneration of Saint Anna (usually known as Saint Anne in English), the name, which by tradition, was assigned to the mother of the Virgin Mary.

In England, this Latin form has been used alongside the vernacular forms Ann and Anne since the late Middle Ages. It was a name that had one pronunciation but many spellings throughout every period of time. But, today, Anna is currently the most common spelling in all English-speaking countries. However, the biblical form of Hannah is presently more popular than all three, but it does have a different sound to it now.

The name Anna has also been the name of the Royals, no matter where they were. It was born by several Russian royals, including an 18th-century sovereign of Russia. However, as perfect as the name is, Anna did not suffice for Mario and Isabel. They knew they needed something more. After all, the name you give your little one will be an everlasting part of their identity, so they picked a name that would pair best with Ana.

The name Sofia means Wisdom and is also of Spanish origin. However, the name, Sofia, is not just restricted to one language. It means astuteness in Greek, which more or less aligns with its Spanish translation. There is a heart-breaking history attached to the name Sofia. It was the name of an early, perhaps mythical, saint who died of grief after her three daughters were killed during the reign of Emperor Hadrian.

Legends about her, her name, and her character arose from a medieval misunderstanding of the phrase "Hagia Sofia," or "Holy Wisdom," which is the name of a large basilica in Constantinople, present-day Istanbul.

This name was common among people who belonged to the continental European Royalty during the Middle Ages. It was later popularized in Britain by the German House of Hanover when they inherited the British throne in the 18th century.

From famous beings in scriptures to characters, people, and film stars, Ana and Sofia are names that have dominated our ears because of how calm and gentle they sound.

For the young couple, these two names together were the epitome of what Anasofia was. Wise and gracious. She was everything this name portrayed and so much more.

Naming their baby Anasofia was a blessing in disguise.

Chapter 4

The Secret Signs

Knowing She Was Special and Different

In this chapter, I want to discuss the importance of listening to your intuition. If you are a mother, a father, or care for someone who recently lost a child, and your gut calls for you to act, this is for you. Intuition is often something we refer to as our sixth sense; it can protect you, it can guide you, and when times are tough, it can support you.

This is how AnaSofia's mother felt. She listened to her intuition – only half of the population have this motherly intuition. It comes into play during birth if a woman feels that something isn't quite right, and sometimes it never leaves you. And, before AnaSofia was even born, her mother knew that she was special.

Of course, all mothers say this about their children. Still, after all these years, it was being in touch with her body and observing her hormonal changes that helped Isabel. Perhaps there was something about the soul the mother ignored, or maybe she was too naive to understand.

I invite all to open their heart and listen to their intuition. If it is somehow to heal your wounds or help someone heal theirs, your intuition will be of great help.

First, we will talk about the general intuition within all of us and, in the end, the motherly one.

The intuitive voice is something we all have. It is how the subconscious mind communicates with the conscious mind. It is a powerful tool, but despite every one of us being blessed with the power of intuition, not everyone can listen to theirs, for it often needs a quiet, calm, reflective environment. To find your way and connect with your intuition, you have to learn to find peace. Once you do, you have to go there when times are complex and listen with all you might to what your heart and soul are telling you because they will always tell you something.

Our intuition wants to guide us, it wants us to do better, and when the journey gets tough, it is always looking out for us. *Always.*

You know the feeling. It is when something within you is speaking to you. It's this feeling of 'knowing,' or for some, it can be a gentle persuasion that something is off, or excellent, or needs our attention through spiritual practices or otherwise. It is subtle and doesn't overpower our conscious mind to gain attention, which is why it can be easily dismissed. Intuition will not come to you, banging at your head. It will be like a silent whisper – enough for you to listen, but quiet that one can easily miss it. The potential is life-changing only if we listen.

It is not to say that people do not doubt the power of intuition because they do. Many skeptics will argue that intuition is pseudoscience when it is not. It is hard for many people to believe that our mind, body, and soul are blessed with this ability to let us know when something is wrong. If it is, then the good thing is science is now on board, and researchers have found the part of the brain where intuition does its brilliant best.

Researchers at Leeds University, after extensive studies, concluded that intuition is not pseudoscience. It is an actual psychological process where the brain uses past experiences and cues from the self and the environment to decide.

Intuition exists in all of us. Whether we believe in it or not is not part of the question, but the more we understand it, the more it can shape our lives for the better. Here is how we can sharpen our intuition to really listen to our thoughts, feeling, and desires, so we know what is ahead.

Always Listen.

Listening: it sounds simple enough. That is because it is. There are no tricks here, no method, no technique, and no skill. All you have to do is shush and give your subconscious mind a chance. Your intuition cannot talk to you if you are not willing to listen. When you start to listen, good things will happen, and your intuition will show you the way.

Never dismiss your gut feeling.

Gut feeling, we have all heard it before, and we all know what it is. The process of trusting your gut is not as simple as the phrase implies. We have all made a decision that we know we should not have made. Even before we made it, our gut guided us not to, yet we still made it, and soon enough, we saw the outcome. So, my advice is never to dismiss your gut. It knows you better than most people.

Feel your feelings.

Intuition is an emotion you can feel. You will feel it when something you choose is right – You will feel it in your belly or your heart. It will send goosebumps down to your skin, a shiver down your spine, or quicken your breath.

Be ready to let bad feelings go.

Negative emotions and negative energy will cloud your judgment and your intuition. Look at it this way; whenever you are angry or depressed, you make rash decisions, and once that anger is gone, you often end up regretting it. So, every time you are about to listen to your intuition, be absolutely sure you are not listening to your vengeful, angry side instead.

Surround yourself with people who bring out the best in you.

It might sound corny, but the people you surround yourself with have an obvious effect on you, your personality, your thoughts, and even your subconscious mind. What they say, how they act, all of it gets fed in our brain, and sometimes the decisions we make in our lives are just a reflection of them. Make sure the people you are hanging out with are those which who you align, not those who clash with your moral and ethical values.

Be mindful of the surroundings.

The more information you can gather from the environment, the more the intuitive, subconscious part of your brain has to work with – and the more accurately it will inform your decisions.

Broaden your horizons.

Sometimes, we feel something about people but cannot quite put the finger on what it is. It can be good or bad, but to become more in tune with what that feeling is, we have to go out and socialize. We have to give time, meaning, and a little thought to our interactions with people. People might be complex; they might seem distant, distracted, and even uninterested at times. The ability to pick up on the thoughts, feelings, and intentions of other people is important. It is called 'empathic accuracy' and, the more time we spend around people, the more we can finely tune our empathic accuracy. That will then sharpen our intuitive abilities.

Find time to be alone.

Being comfortable in your solitude gives you the time, the understanding, and the chance to know yourself better. It also allows you to tune in to your intuition. By focusing on yourself, you give your mind a chance to wander and be open to what comes to you. No matter what it may be: feelings, thoughts, or words.

This feeling of solitude will help you get rid of mental clutter, and hopefully, it will make way for you to be in tune with your intuition.

Your intuition can get trapped in your dreams.

When you close your eyes and fall asleep, your brain does not sleep with you. Instead, it sends you off to a land where your brain is free to make up scenarios and live a life it truly wants. Dreams require no reasoning, logic, meditation, or processing of thoughts or investigation but, it requires support from your mind. The things you dream about are not just limited to wishful thinking; most times, they are more than that. Our dreams mirror our subconscious mind, and sometimes our deepest and darkest thoughts are expressed through them. Only if we pay attention to the tiny details can we find our guiding light.

The awakening that we all crave can be filled if only we give our intuitive abilities a chance. Since it is powerful, it can shed light so we can know the truth. Sometimes it can lead to unique insights because they are always sending us warnings and encouragement. Often, we are too busy to notice. However, just like everything else, intuition has its pros and cons, so it doesn't mean you should follow it blindly. It is still important to use common sense and a balance of rationality. It would help if you had a balance of both – call into play both the intuitive and rational parts of the brain to position yourself to reach the best decisions. Trusting your intuition might be difficult at first if you're not used to it but give it time and trust it bit by bit if that feels better. It will be worth it.

Luckily, our intuition is so deeply instinctual that even if we've been out of touch with it for our entire lives, it is still there inside of us, waiting for us to summon its wisdom.

Motherly Intuition.

A mother's intuition is perhaps just a small part of that entire spiritual experience of motherhood…

Mothers are highly intuitive. That is a fact that even doctors and scientists acknowledge. There have been enough documented cases of mothers intuitively knowing when their children are in trouble, even if far away. So many times, mothers have felt a strong urge to reach out to their children and followed the instinct to find their child in trouble. At times mothers have been proven right when they insisted something was wrong with their child's health, despite an all-clear from doctors.

Though the veracity of a mother's intuition has been proven many times, nobody can say how or why it works. It is almost like a mother is nudged or prompted that her child needs help. In an online survey, ninety-six percent of mothers admitted they have had intuitions that turned out to be right about their children's welfare.

I believe a mother is intuitive because she is inextricably linked to her child as a result of the birth connection. When she gives birth to the child, only the physical link gets severed with the umbilical cord. In every other way, she stays connected and responsible for the welfare and upbringing of the little life she has brought into the world. That is what gives her the strength, depths of love, sympathy, forgiveness, and understanding that mothers are known for.

And so, mothers learn to be better humans through the experience of motherhood. They become almost spiritual beings through the deep love and protection they feel for their children. And when they get a sixth sense about their child, there is no question about finding the courage or confidence to follow the gut feel through. Their overpowering love gives them that.

A mother's intuition is perhaps just a small part of that entire spiritual experience of motherhood... It is without a doubt that Isabel felt this motherly instinct. If you feel it, treasure it and love it as it grows and guides you through happiness and not-so-happy days.

Chapter 5

The Day She Was Born
The Joys the Shock

The birth of a child is one of the happiest days in a parent's life. It is a feeling like no other, and no words in the English language or any other language can describe what it feels like. When Anasofia was born, Isabel and Mario went through the same emotions. However, with their angel's birth, they soon realized that their angel indeed was special – unique in a way that would require an extra bit of attention.

Anasofia was born with an extra chromosome, and it took a long time for Mario and Isabel to understand what it was. If this is your case and your baby has an extra love chromosome: do not worry; it is natural for parents of babies with any syndrome. You will experience shock, sadness, and fear, and that is okay. The world is scary, and the unknown and hidden difficulties of raising a child with intellectual and developmental disabilities can cause stress in many new parents but don not be disappointed. It is not your fault, and despite the disability your child is living with, be assured that your child can lead a healthy and everyday life. Veteran parents have a comforting message for all new parents out there: do not worry; it is overwhelming, but it will get better. So, so, so much better. Never give up and consider every day a blessing.

If you are struggling, here are some recommendations I would like to share with you for the early stages after learning your child has a syndrome.

Medical professionals mean well, but they can still say the wrong things.

Doctors are human beings. They are trained professionals who are aware of the workings of the human body. However, some of them still need help with forming the right words, especially when it comes to giving not-so-good news. I wish I had realized this sooner; I wish I had realized that the doctor who delivered our child and diagnosed her did not understand the beauty of raising a child with special needs.

He was not rude, but his words were not too comforting. He was blunt, straightforward, and almost too distant from the situation, but that is not his fault. Maybe being in a hospital made him like this. I wish I would not have let the harshness of his words affect me in such a profound way. I wish I could go back in time and reassure myself that he meant well. When he saw my angel as differently abled, I saw wonderment. Where he saw delays and disability, I saw triumphs. Where he saw pain, I saw love. AnaSofia's parents thought she was perfect.

Your child's syndrome does not mean they would have to sacrifice life.

Being diagnosed with a syndrome is not a death sentence. It's something a lot of people have grown to think- but it's not true. A parent raising a child with down syndrome recalled her experience with her child: "When my daughter was born, I wish I had known that things would be OK — that we would laugh a lot and that she would bring me so much joy every day."

This life can be a blessing.

If you go on the internet, you will see a lot of parents talk about how before their child with special needs arrived, their lives were chaotic, fast, and extremely stressful. But with their child's birth, it was a sign from the universe to slow down and appreciate the beauty of life. That comes from the road less traveled. If your child gets to live their life for one minute to anywhere in adulthood it is always a blessing.

Your baby is still your baby.

Your baby is not defined by the syndrome or special needs. Yes, your child has issues and is different, but they will still remain a unique little person with a personality of their own. They will have likes and dislikes, strengths and weaknesses just like everyone. Your child will have mood swings; they will jump on trends and stereotypes, surprise you and delight you, also make you mad and disappointed — just the same as every child. They are still your child. If you love them and give them the attention they deserve, you will soon see that.

Do not, even for a moment, think your child is a curse.

You may or may not have other children; if you do, it is a possibility other parents might scare you that your special angel can become a troubling presence for them, but that is not true. The opposite is more likely.

It is wise to let your other children know what's going on.

Your children will learn with time that their brother or sister is a little different and that means you will need to pay them special attention. It is completely natural to be involved in this one child, and maybe without realizing it, we can be fussing so much on our child with special needs that we forget to check in on our other kids and their needs. However, that is the one thing we have to avoid, and that will only happen when you sit down and have the talk with your children.

Shed positive light on the life of children with any syndrome.

This is the experience of another parent:

Within hours after learning that my son had Down syndrome, I thought about all the things any parent would think about. My mind raced with the thought of the future, and I was terrified for my son. I was terrified that he could be ostracized or bullied in school.

I thought back to the time I was in school, I realized that we barely saw kids with special abilities, let alone Down syndrome, and we really didn't know anything about them. It made me realize that awareness is the most important thing for a bright future. When people know that children like my son exist, they'll know that it's not unusual; instead, they will treat them with the care and attention they require.

I am glad we live in a world that's learning what down syndrome is now – one where my son can walk in hallways and not be greeted with laughs and insults but a world with hi-fives and hugs.

Your Child is a Typical Kid.

Of course, when one says typical kid, they do not mean it in the average fashion. Children with any syndrome have their own quirks, just like every other child does, and the way they feel is just the way that a typical kid would. They have the ability to do everything normally, provided that we keep our minds and hearts open to their ways.

They understand you and your ways, so take some time and understand theirs, and you will find yourself amazed at their ability to express.

Non-Verbality Can Break Your Heart.

Children with any syndrome are not usually verbal with the way they feel and things that they understand. This can cause them to be angry, frustrated, and sometimes even upset because, just like every child, they feel things too. If they have a bad day at school, they might not be able to come up to you and rant to you about it verbally, but they will use their unique ways of communication, Unfortunately, that can include getting physical or screaming.

Understand them at that time and know that whenever they are behaving in a way that might not be favorable, they are trying to tell you something. They are trying to tell you that they are upset and need to express themselves. We, as parents, need to try to figure it out for them, and there is no easy way to do it. It is a long process, and you might have to mend your ways, but know that while your heart breaks at their non-verbality, theirs is trying to communicate something. For this, expression through music or paintings can work well.

Kids with Syndromes Love Teenage Years!

Being lovable and sweet comes naturally to kids with any syndrome. However, they are not always up for your love through cuddles, hugs, and other forms of affection. Well, doesn't that sound like every teenager running away from their parents when they try and hug them? That is just how children with syndrome feel. Not all, but a significant portion of them do. Some might send the classic teenage stink-eye your way as a teenager, while others might accept a hug or two.

They have their own set of emotions, just like their typical teenage peers, and we need to acknowledge those as parents while we take joy in every emotion they feel and every form of expression they send our way.

Stages Too Shall Pass.

For children with syndromes, there will be stages that might make things difficult for you as a parent. This could include their potty-training stage, and more importantly, the running-away stage when they would run and run, and you will just find yourself chasing them. This happens more often within the age bracket of 5-8 and can vary from child to child. However, as parents, you must know and believe that they do grow out of it.

Once they grow out of it, you grow out of it, and it passes. These stages, or phases, do not stay forever, so always believe that it will pass to make it easier for you to act on it.

Your child will not be a Child forever.

Parents might want to treat their children with special needs like younger children, but we must understand that they will become teenagers, adults, and then people of their own. We need to support them in getting older, better, and more responsible instead of continuing to treat them like children. Our children are not in the Man Child category for sure. They have adult goals and adult responsibilities just like any other adult do.

Be sure to let your child feel their age. If they are in their teenage years, treat them like a teenager. If they are growing adults ready to graduate college, treat them like it. It is said that children are always babies to their parents, no matter how old they are, but we as parents need to also understand that your baby has come into this world with a purpose and goal of their own, and we must encourage that instead of covering bases for them because we think they aren't capable.

New Languages Come Your Way.

With children who have syndromes comes a world of their own. It is a world that we parents need to be well-acquainted with. This world has a language of its own, and this language has quite a lot of new words as well as acronyms that you have to befriend. These include IFSP, IEP, PT, ST, OT, OHS, VSD, and trust me – the list could go on and on.

As parents, you will find yourself learning new things every day, and this unique language is something that will come your way. It might be challenging to embrace the intricacies of this new language, but with time you will understand the beauty, as well as the efficiency of these acronyms, for your life as a parent.

You Will Master the Art of Problem-Solving.

We all know it is not easy. We all know that sometimes, things happen around us that we do not know how to react to, and perhaps no book or tutorial can teach us. There will be situations where the solutions will come only from within you and the relationship that you share with your child, and that, my friends, makes you the master of problem-solving!

Community of Parents like You.

The extra chromosome is going to be the binding factor between you and many other parents like myself. The system of a community, in this case, can be incredibly helpful as you can share ideas on expression for your children, along with the best educational and employment opportunities.

More than anything else, you will find people going through the same struggles as you, and when that happens, a significant amount of your emotional build-up is taken care of. If you have someone to talk to, who understands just what you are going through, it is indeed a blessing!

Not Your Quintessential Happy Endings.

By far, we have established that where having a child with an extra chromosome can be a beautiful experience of its own, we cannot let go of the realities attached with the extra chromosome. In the world that we live in, it is highly possible that your special child might not get what they deserve or have to go through struggles because you have been unaware of so many things, but it will pass. Your happy ending might not be the way that you had imagined for it to be or come your way when you wanted it the most but hang in there. Trust me when I say it. It will come to you eventually.

YOU Are Important Too.

Being able to cope with a child with special needs can be exhausting. It can physically as well as mentally exhaust us. It is natural, but it doesn't have to be perpetual. Not for you, not for your partner, and not for your friend in the community you have built. Be sure to take good care of yourself to make sure you are okay, and so are the ones you love with all your heart.

We must ensure that we are taken care of in every aspect, be it sleep, nutrition or exercise. It will only make things easier for our loved ones and us.

It is Their Life.

Most of us find ourselves drowning in the deep oceans of love, care, affection, and protection that we want to reflect upon our children, particularly the ones with special needs however, we must understand that down the road.

Eventually, when your child is grown enough, they will want to lead their lives their way.

Once you create a path for them, they will want to walk it on their own. They will have their struggles, their achievements, their friends and relationships, and everything that they need they will have. You will have to step back and watch them take over the world as their accomplice sometimes, and sometimes, as their cheerleaders.

Even though AnaSofia's life was short, her parents always envisioned her school, her friends, and in general her life. After her passing every year, her mom would meditate and recreate her life as it would be that year. This mental and spiritual exercise also brought her great peace.

Chapter 6

Her Days in This Realm

Her Life at Home

Ever wondered what the definition of being truly selfless is? Well, if you have had a child with special needs or know someone in close capacity who has a child with special needs in their home, you have an idea. There is absolutely no denying the fact that taking care of a baby or a young adult with special needs is nothing but the absolute and true definition of selfless and sincere love. Many people argue that it is hard, and it is something that takes a lot out of you, and while that is true, it is also an incredibly rewarding feeling.

I can say that with full confidence because taking care of Anasofia was an absolute privilege and wonder. It wasn't just a privilege for me but also for the entire family that found themselves associated with her. The love, experience, and affection we shared for her were calming and brought us all together. In no way does that mean that it was a breezy experience. It was rough, and when I talk about things being rough, I want to tell you that there were times that things only got rougher because I did not have anyone to tell me it was going to be that way.

Things got difficult with time, be it feeding her, cleaning her, bathing her, or just generally trying to teach her some of the basics of life. With this set of difficulties came a set of relief as well. That relief often came in the face of her smile. Of course, it sounds like a utopian idea to be in a problem and then in peace the very next second, but all of us who have been through it are well-aware of how possible that is.

The key through all of this is to make sure that whatever you do, you do it with unconditional love and affection. More so, it would help if you comprehended that completely none of this your fault. However, it is something that is now part of your life, and you need to make certain changes to your lifestyle to ensure a comfortable living for everyone involved. One way to move in that direction is always to consider physical therapy. It is incredibly important, and physical therapy like massages can help you and your child alike.

More things that are advised from my end would be to learn how to use oxygen machines, cardio-respiratory techniques, and other techniques that could save you the constant need to be around a medical professional or need medical help. The idea of having to always be in touch with a medical professional can also be incredibly tiring, and if learning a few things could save you that, then it is seriously advised.

Where things will get tough, know that you are strong and should not be afraid of handling all these things around you. After all, your special needs children are just unique, that is all. They are unique, just like every other child, and they are amazingly loving babies. Because of Anasofia, my family grew in ways that we never imagined or envisioned. My world changed, and it changed in some of the best ways I could have wanted. There were issues and concerns, and I am not going to sugarcoat the experience, but at the end of the day, it was something that required patience, and if you are patient in a situation like this, the rewards are more heartwarming than you could ever imagine.

In all of this and more, my recommendation would be simple. It would be to love and accept the life of the children with special needs. They have needs that they need your help with, and as a parent and caregiver, you must ensure you take care of as many of them as you can. Yes, it is incredibly difficult to avoid problems and to remain out of shock after having a child with special needs. It is not easy, but you must know that you are not alone. I personally recommend the parents that they take therapy or enroll themselves in special schools where the parents as well as the special needs child.

I say it is absolutely integral because there must be no compromise on the social integration of the child and their parents. These places, be it schools or therapy organizations, tend to create a better environment for everyone involved. It allows stimulation and creates a sense of learning followed by practice at home. In the times that we live in, there is a certain amount of awareness in regard to any syndrome as well as mental illnesses that the parents might find themselves drowning in. And that means there is always a solution waiting for us once we decide that we no longer want to be ashamed or hide from what is our reality.

We have talked about what needs to be done when there is a special child around you but let us talk in detail about what a special needs child really is. A special needs child is a youth who has been determined to require special attention and specific necessities that other children do not. The state may declare this status for the purpose of offering benefits and assistance for the child's well-being and growth. Special needs can also be a legal designation, particularly in the adoption and foster care community, wherein the child and guardian receive support to help them both lead productive lives.

The basic understanding here is that the definition of special needs pertaining to a child includes a wide variety of conditions, including physical ailments, learning disabilities, and terminal illness. More so, parents and guardians of special needs children usually receive tax credits or deductions to help offset the cost of raising a special needs child. Some special needs children are able to go to public schools that offer a wide range of educational and emotional support programs, like occupational therapy and one-on-one teacher aides in the classroom.

The assistance and medical attention that may be required to elevate the quality of life for special needs children can result in long-term and escalating costs. The extent of the child's condition may call for far-reaching medical support to allow the child to live and thrive. For example, a child with a debilitating or life-threatening condition that is permanent could require constant medical support throughout their lives. There is no other option but for us to provide that help and care for that child.

They may need to be monitored on a regular basis in case their ailments become exacerbated. Support equipment may be needed to provide the child with mobility around the residence, and the procurement of support animals such as specially trained dogs may be needed. The idea of therapy dogs has always proved to be beneficial for children with illnesses, particularly illnesses that fall into the paradigm of Down Syndrome. That extra chromosome does require some extra effort on the parents, the society they form, and the medical practitioners involved in the process. If you are looking to make that effort, then rest assured, you will bear the fruit of the same.

A special needs child may have a life-threatening condition, or they may have severe learning disabilities. Either way, it is a child that requires special attention and care that other children do not receive. It might sound harsh, but that is what it is, and that is what needs to be done.

Certain considerations need to be taken care of in this regard. These considerations include certain things. A special needs child may require alternative approaches to education that accommodate their conditions and work toward creating ways for them to further their capacity to learn and develop. These could be special schools that are now easily accessible to many people from bigger cities. I do understand that it might be a problem for many who live in smaller towns. The good news is that the internet is an outstanding resource for your babies and yourself. There is so much information and education that can be learned on the internet, it is phenomenal.

This education will train the children in the best possible ways, keeping in mind their unique problems and concerns. For instance, a child with impaired physical mobility or challenges communicating through traditional verbal cues may need to be trained in other ways, and they may also need training in how to apply those skills in the classroom and real-world settings. It is appallingly amazing to know that even if you do not have physical access to these facilities, the internet and smart devices have created a world for you to access and own.

In instances where a special needs child has cognitive impairments, their education may require expertise in addressing such issues and finding methods to connect with them. Some examples of this can include taking substantially more time and effort to ensure they can understand the lesson and advance to another stage of learning. All of these can happen in person or online, which can work particularly well due to the coronavirus pandemic. The pandemic has impacted more children and young adults, and with that more online learning opportunities have sprung up.

These opportunities include those for children with special needs. You could be in a remote town in Ohio and still have access to Los Angeles' best school for children with special needs. With time, inclusion will come. We have to wait for it. The process of inclusion has started on many different fronts, the completion of it awaits.

Keep in mind that your babies are not your difficulties but a way to make you stronger. They want your love, affection, and attention as much as you can give them. When you live with them, you tend to get frustrated and sometimes even lose hope but always understand and remember that these ideas are temporary and the smile on your baby's face is permanent.

Chapter 7

Grieving the Loss of a Child

The Family and Her Soul

Death is a grim word. It is an event that changes an individual forever. It tends to create a void within people, and sometimes, the void is so deep that it can barely be dealt with. For many, this void is not visible up until a situation comes up, and they fall into this deep void, with absolutely no way up. All hopes, faith, and desires come crashing down like a huge ball of ice in a deadly avalanche. This does not quite sound like something that one could prepare themselves for. It is true. Death is inevitable.

Anasofia's parents knew it. Their doctors had warned them. One day she will stop living. And so, it happened. After spending days at her great grandparents' house where all the family was gathered, she stopped breathing and passed away. This day was a sad day for all her family. The hardest and most excruciating day ever. She stopped beathing and her heart stopped as well. She cried a little as if she was saying goodbye and one second later, she was asleep looking peacefully.

This death hits us even harder when it is our child – someone who was created out of our flesh and was the apple of our eyes. It is almost as if with the loss of a child comes the loss of a parent as well. Parents tend to lose parts of themselves and knowing that the loss will never be compensated for, can be even more painful. However, the parents, especially those who lose a child with special needs, must know that no parent is prepared for the death of their child. Parents are simply not supposed to outlive their children; that is what the cycle of life tells us. In this case, it becomes essential for the parent to know that grieving is a process, and it is one that they need to live.

It is important to remember that how long your child lived does not determine the size of your loss; it can be just as hurtful at any age. Many things change with death, especially since parents of young children are intimately involved in their daily lives. Death changes every aspect of family life, often leaving an enormous emptiness. This is the case with children with special needs because of how much involvement the parents need to have in their life for them to lead a better life.

The death of older children or adolescents, too, is difficult because children at this age are beginning to reach their potential and become independent individuals. More so, when an adult child dies, you lose not only a child but often a close friend, a link to grandchildren, and an irreplaceable source of emotional and practical support. You may find that you also grieve for the hopes and dreams you had for your child. It is not just the child who leaves you; it is an entire life you had imagined that gets shaken up.

All the potential that will never be realized, the experiences that you will never share, and the life milestones that you will not be able to accompany them to, will all hauntingly come to you after their death. Things can get even worse for people who lose their only child. They might feel stripped of their identity of being parents. The pain will always be part of the parent, regardless of when and how they lost their child. Absurdly enough, the silver lining is that time hides, if not heals everything.

With time, most parents find a way forward and begin experiencing happiness and meaning in life once again. What I want to tell you all is that this phase does come. In my experience, the pain always remains within you, but somehow, you find the courage to move on and resume your life. Maybe it is the strength that your angel sends from above, but somehow and somewhere, that strength becomes a part of you. Take your time to grieve, but know that eventually, life will move on, and to catch up, you might have to, as well.

Make sure that you grieve through all of this. Whatever grief reaction you have is valid. Grief reactions after the death of a child are often similar to those after other losses. But they are often more intense and last longer. Many grief reactions include intense shock, confusion, disbelief, denial, overwhelming sadness and despair, extreme guilt, anger, feelings of bitterness, loneliness, resentment, losing faith, isolation, and more. All of these emotions that topple your thought process sometimes put you in a position where doing the daily chores can become a hassle.

Although grief is always profound when a child dies, some parents tend to have an especially difficult time. Even as time passes, the grief remains intense, and they feel it is impossible to return to normal life. Some parents may even think about hurting themselves to escape from the pain. Everyone grieves differently, and they have all the right to. In fact, the timings of the grief reaction also varies.

Some people expect that grief should be resolved over a specific time, such as a year or maybe even two. But this is not true. The initial severe and intense grief that you feel will not be continuous or consistent. Pain will come and go, and over time, your grief may come in waves that are gradually less intense and less frequent. Even years after a child's death, important events and milestones in the lives of other children can trigger grief. Significant days such as graduations, weddings, or the first day of a new school year are common triggers. At these times, you may find yourself thinking about how old your child would be or what they would look like or be doing if still alive.

Now, let us discuss the differences in how different parents grieve. Parents may grieve differently depending on their gender and their daily role in a child's life. One parent may find that talking helps, while the other may need quiet time to grieve alone. Cultural expectations and role differences also affect how parents grieve. Men are often expected to control their emotions, be strong, and take charge of the family. Women may be expected to cry openly and want to talk about their grief.

If you are a working parent, you may become more involved in your job to escape the sadness and daily reminders at home. A stay-at-home parent may be surrounded by constant reminders and may feel a lack of purpose now that their job as a caregiver has abruptly ended. This is especially true for a parent who spent months or even years caring for a child with cancer.

Differences in grieving can cause relationship difficulties when parents need each other's support the most. One parent may believe that the other is not grieving properly, or that a lack of open grief means they did not love their child. Talk openly about your grief with your partner. Work to understand and accept each other's coping styles. It can help you because you need to accept that the child is gone at the end of the day. Now the parents have to rely on each other for love, support, and emotional assistance.

Where parents are often the focus of attention when a child dies, the grief of their siblings tends to get overshadowed sometimes. It is essential to understand that they too have lost a significant person, and the change in the home environment impacts them severely. The death of a sibling is a tremendous loss for a child: they lose a family member, a confidant, and a life-long friend. If your child died of prolonged sickness, all the attention has been on that child, while the other might have gotten neglected in the process.

Parents, while grieving, can also take care of their other surviving children. They can do this through the following ways:

- Make grief a shared family experience. Include children in discussions about memorial plans.

- Spend as much time as possible with your children, talking about their siblings or playing together.

- Make sure children understand that they are not responsible for a sibling's death. Help them let go of regrets and guilt.

- Never compare siblings to your child who died. Make sure your child knows that you don't expect them to "fill in" for the child who passed.

- Set reasonable limits on their behavior. But try not to be either overprotective or overly permissive. It is normal to feel protective of surviving children.

- Ask a close family member or friend to spend extra time with siblings if your grief prevents you from giving them the attention they need.

This will help the other children the parents have, but there is a lot that parents can do to help their own grieving process. As much as it hurts, it is incredibly natural to grieve, and the following suggestions might help.

- Talk about your child often and use their name.

- Ask family and friends for help with housework, errands, and caring for other children. This will give you important time to think, remember, and grieve.

- Take time deciding what to do with your child's belongings. Do not rush to pack up your child's room or to give away toys and clothes.

- Prepare ahead of time for how to respond to difficult questions like, "How many children do you have?" Or comments like, "At least you have other children." Remember that people are not trying to hurt you; they just do not know what to say.

- Prepare for how you want to spend significant days, such as your child's birthday or the anniversary of your child's death. You may want to spend the day looking at photos and sharing memories or start a family tradition, such as planting flowers.

- Because of the intensity and isolation of parental grief, parents may benefit from a support group where they can share their experiences with other parents who understand their grief and can offer hope.

See, I could say many helpful things right now, and none of those could make sense to a parent who has lost someone they loved. Everyone has their own process of grieving, but the matter remains that one should expect that they will never really get over the death of a child as it is a loss that is irreplaceable and kills a part of you. However, they will learn to live with this loss, making this loss a part of who they are. There might be a shift in priorities, meaning of life, and so much more, and where it could be difficult, maybe even seem impossible, happiness and purpose will find you eventually!

For some parents, an important step may be creating a legacy for their child. You may choose to honor your child by volunteering at a local hospital or a support organization. Or you may work to support interests your child once had, start a memorial fund or plant trees in your child's memory. It is important to remember that it is never disloyal to your child to reengage in life and enjoy new experiences.

Each of your children changes your life. They show you new ways to love, new things to find joy in and new ways to look at the world. A part of each child's legacy is that the changes they bring to your family continue after death. The memories of joyful moments you spent with your child and the love you shared will live on and always be part of you.

Grieve the way you wish but try your best not to let that grief take you down. I lost a child, and I almost thought that I was done. I found a way, and I promise you that if you hang in there, you will find your way too.

Anasofia's memorial was a sad day but also full of love and family support.

Chapter 8

Days After

The Family and the Friends Journey

Grief is weird. There, I said it. None of us know what the right or wrong way to grieve might be, as all of us have figured our own ways out to express the sadness that comes our way, especially with the loss of a loved one. While some might deal with the loss of their child well, owing to a lot of support and love from friends and family, some might need their time. I am trying to make here that no matter what someone tells you about grief, you must know that any way of grieving as long as it doesn't hurt you is entirely alright.

Our Anasofia was the core of our hearts, and when she left, our grieving was immense. However, how we dealt with that grief shaped us as people for the rest of our lives, and quite honestly, it has only gotten better. Let us talk about the sorrow and grief we feel and what we can do as allies to help someone going through it. It can be difficult for us to help others if we do not know what they are going through. After all, we cannot learn how to help a grieving friend without objectively knowing what their experience may be. Let us take a closer look at grief, what it will look like for specific individuals, and when it may become something more concerning.

The last chapter discussed grief and death in detail for the person going through it. It is time to talk about how people around us can help us grieve better. This is for anyone who has people around them with misery surrounding them. This is for anyone who wants to be an ally to all of those in pain. It could be an incredibly fulfilling experience to be an ally in this case.

First things first, let us understand grief briefly again. Grief is the process that we go through when we experience a significant loss in our lives. This may result from the loss of someone close to us (which is often referred to when we mention grief) or the loss of something essential to us, like a job. When we experience grief, we will usually go through an extended period of sadness and other emotions as we yearn for that which we have lost. The duration of this grief will be different for every individual, but the feelings will often fade over time. The question comes down to: what can you do?

1. Reach out regularly.

The days and weeks immediately following a loss can be the most difficult. It is during this time that many will provide the most support. However, this initial support may lose momentum over time. One of the most important tips to remember if you are looking to provide support is to reach out regularly. Although your friend may feel over-whelmed or withdrawn at times, knowing that they have someone to turn to when they need it is a significant relief. Whether you choose to reach out every other day or every week, stick to a regular schedule and let them know that you are there for them. Questions like: *How are you holding up? How are you doing this week?*

2. Find ways to help your friend out as they navigate the grieving process.

Providing emotional support is typically the main focus of people looking to help their friends through grief. However, this is not the only way you can offer support. You can also help out a grieving friend by doing things they may not feel up to doing. For example, you can offer to do little things like make a meal for them or take out the trash. These small gestures mean a lot to those who are grieving.

Additionally, it can reduce some of the stress they are feeling as they attempt to get back to daily life. If you live nearby and you can, consider helping your friend in this way. Questions like: *Is There Anything I Can Do for You? Do you need anything?*

3. Listen more than you speak.

We all have different experiences when it comes to grief. This is because our loss and the circumstances surrounding it will vary greatly. The way that we cope with this loss will also be different from how others cope with it. Because of these variables, it can be challenging for us to provide the right advice to others. The solution? Rather than trying to do this, take a listening approach, and be the person to whom they vent their feelings. If they ask for advice, you may want to tell them about your personal experience. Otherwise, you can let them know that while you do not have the answer, you are willing to figure it out with them. Just be there for them. Phrases like, *"I'm Here for You"* can go miles.

4. Do fun things that will help take your friend's mind away from their grief.

We all have to deal with our emotions to get through them. That said, we all want a break from our feelings sometimes. One great way to support your friend is to act as that escape for them when they are feeling overwhelmed. You can do fun things with them, like spending the day together, going out for lunch or dinner, seeing a movie, or even just spending time at their house. No matter what you choose to do, it can be helpful for your friend to have a way to get their mind off of their loss. This can also build the relationship between you two so that they know they can feel safe opening up to you when they need to do so. You can always ask them things like, *"Would you like to go somewhere or do something today?"*

5. Give your friend space if they ask for it.

Giving support to those who are not feeling their best is always a great thing to do. However, you have to understand that some people may feel overwhelmed at times. Rather than welcoming the support they usually would, they may want to be left alone to work through their thoughts. Some people may take this as their friends not wanting help, but this may not be true. Instead, please give them the space that they need until they feel ready to socialize again. Just because they are not ready now does not mean they will not need your support in the future. It might not feel like it, but sometimes space is integral. Always be understanding of that and get used to using terms like, *"That's okay. I will reach back out to you later!"*

6. Get professional help.

Another essential thing to remember when you're looking to provide support for a grieving friend is that we may not always be able to give the proper support. Their close friends and family will be a significant source of support during this time. While we can listen and be there for them, they may need professional help to get through some of their more complicated feelings. If they are dealing with severe grief or depression, one way to help them is to suggest seeing a counselor.

For the most part, people will have counseling resources near them. If your friend manages to find a counselor near them that they connect to, that is excellent. With that in mind, it may not be easy to find the right resources in a given area. If your friend is having trouble seeking out help, you may want to consider online counseling.

7. Volunteer you time.

People who have dealt with dead family members firsthand often want to support others with that. Whether you are a grief survivor or care for someone who has, you have valuable experience to help others. Becoming a volunteer makes a difference in a person's life. It also positively affects your own life.

Volunteering offers different rewards for everyone. Many volunteers say sharing their time makes them feel good. They also say it helps them build new friendships and widens their support network.

There are various ways to get started. Once you have decided to become a volunteer, think about your interests, strengths, and areas of expertise. Consider how you could use these to help organizations with their missions. Service and support. Awareness and education. Fundraising. Advocacy. There is so much that can happen if we choose for it to.

8. Write a letter to them.

If counseling is something that you do not see yourself suggesting, you could write to them and make them feel better about the situation they are going through. Here is a letter that can be customized accordingly for a family member or friend who recently found themselves grieving, particularly at the loss of a child.

This brief letter is for parents who have suffered the death of a child recently. I hope this can become an ointment to help heal your wound.

You are not alone, you are loved, and you are a great parent.

Many can relate to you and your family's experience or link to some of the trauma you may have suffered.

I understand that nothing can cure the hurt you are going through, but trust that this, at least, can become an ointment to help heal your scar. Please see below some words of encouragement. Perhaps it can help you get through the struggles of grief. This letter is to let you know you will be fine and that you are courageous and strong.

The letter could be a part of what could be done by allies in this case. These allies are more often people who have dealt with grief themselves. Either way, it is essential to know that being there for someone makes a huge difference.

Here is a little prayer for the ones in grief. Your child's legacy will live on, and it will live in through you. May you have peace and patience with the process that you have!

Chapter 9

The Years After

Her Legacy

"You will lose someone you can't live without, and your heart will be badly broken, and the bad news is that you never completely get over the loss of your beloved. But this is also the good news. They live forever in your broken heart that doesn't seal back up. And you come through. It's like having a broken leg that never heals perfectly—that still hurts when the weather gets cold, but you learn to dance with the limp."

— Anne Lamott

They say family is everything. And they are right. This is not something many people realize; they lose someone incredibly dear to them. One who was part of their family and made their lives light up by just being a part of it. When this family member leaves them, they understand that it is not just painful but downright excruciating. The same people who had dealt with one or more dead family members firsthand often want to support others in times of similar grief. They always want to help, and that is also the effort that counts.

"When someone you love dies, and you're not expecting it, you don't lose her all at once; you lose her in pieces over a long time—the way the mail stops coming, and her scent fades from the pillows and even from the clothes in her closet and drawers. Gradually, you accumulate the parts of her that are gone. Just when the day comes—when there's a particular missing part that overwhelms you with the feeling that she's gone, forever— there comes another day, and another specifically missing part."

— John Irving, A Prayer for Owen Meany

Whether you are a grief survivor or care for someone who has been one, you have valuable experience to help others. Becoming a volunteer makes a difference in a person's life. It also positively affects their own life. This volunteering, in a way, is the reason that society works as it does. People, who understand people and have empathy run the show of the world, and well, what better empathetic gestures than to be with someone grieving a significant loss like that of their child?

"The purpose of life is not to be happy. It is to be useful, to be honorable, to be compassionate, to have it make some difference that you have lived and lived well."

— Ralph Waldo Emerson

Now, volunteering offers different rewards for everyone. In fact, many volunteers say sharing their time makes them feel good. They also say it helps them build new friendships and widens their support network. Through the course of the book, we have discussed the importance of support groups and how they can help overcome grief in the best possible way. There are, however, ways to go about this in general.

The question comes down to how can a volunteer help? Of course, people want to help, but a lot of times, the problem comes in when they do not know how to take the lead on trying to help others. Let us take a look at a few ways that one can get started on making a difference in this case and more. The thing is that once you have decided that you want to become a volunteer, think about all your interests, strengths, and areas of expertise.

> *"The purpose of life is to contribute in some way to making things better."*

> — Robert F. Kennedy

You could begin with considering how you could use these to help organizations or even people with their needs and missions in this regard. There are quite a few ways that these things can be looked at. Here are some examples.

- **Service and Support.**

Some programs provide information and help people with grief, loss, and primarily, death. There are several ways that they offer help. The first would be telephone hotlines.

More often than not, the use of these hotlines is commercialized, and people can always reach out to them. They can also be, and often are, available round the clock. The second support program could be proper support groups. Many families that have been grieving lead support groups for people suffering from the same. This holds particularly true for people who have children with special needs.

- **Awareness and Education.**

This is one of the best options that people have. Organizations often need people to help raise awareness and educate others about special needs children who struggle and the families involved. They may also provide tips about having a healthy coping mechanism after loss and offer follow-up care after the treatment ends. It could be happening through presentations at schools, workplaces, or even health fairs. With the Coronavirus pandemic being such a determining factor in decisions made and events held, these could very well also be happening online. You can help by learning how to teach a session about children with special needs and the grief surrounding the very conclusion in many cases.

These sessions could be at your workplace, community centers, or even places of worship. There are many people who have faith and who believe in their respective churches. They can always be addressed, and awareness can be raised on a fundamental level while also impacting a large number of people in the process. Different services in this process could include providing services at local organizations with event planning or even joining a committee that plans new

- **Fundraising.**

Fundraising always helps. Organizations usually need to raise money to maintain services and programs for people struggling to cope with grief and their families. If you want to help, you can always consider getting involved in fundraising activities, such as races, golf tournaments, luncheons, dinners, plays, concerts, fashion shows, auctions, and many other things. You can also donate money to research platforms regarding special needs and mental wellness about coping with grief and trauma.

- **Advocacy.**

When one talks about advocacy, they are looking at supporting and speaking in favor of a specific cause. In this case, and in accordance with this book's very reason, advocating the cause of special needs, the attention is required, and the post-care mechanisms for families who go through pain, grief, and absolute misery in many ways. This could very well involve supporting laws that help people and their families. Or, it may include speaking out about issues that affect people with cancer. You can also help lead an effort to change policies around access to healthcare, mental health, or even funding for research.

These things can be done to make sure that you are doing your best to help people around you. However, these were things on a broader spectrum. There are usually opportunities in your local area to offer help.

Here are ways to find volunteer opportunities in your local area:

- Tell your family, friends, coworkers, and health care providers that you want to get involved in volunteer activities. Talk with them about your interests and ways you may want to help. Ask for their ideas about how you can volunteer.

- Find out about local volunteer programs where you live. Contact your local hospital, cancer center, associations, and places of worship to learn about their health volunteer programs. Ask how you can become involved. You can also look for announcements in your local newspaper, library, and community center. Or check the social media sites of organizations in your community.

In and through all of this, social media will always remain a key component. Anyone looking to help can always and must always take help from social media. This could help them find better options regarding places they could donate to, volunteer at, and more. Grief needs service. The more people can come out and support it, the better it will be for everyone in society.

Chapter 10

Not Letting Go

Keeping Her Memory

"Grief is not...a 'two steps forward, one step backward' kind of journey; it is often one step forward, two steps in a circle, one step backward. It takes time, patience, and, yes, lots of backward motion before forward motion occurs."

— Dr. Alan Wolfelt

Memories are meant to be kept. If they were not, they would not be called memories. When AnaSofia passed, I always had support. I consider myself incredibly lucky to have the kind of support that I did. I talked about it to people around me. However, sometimes I wonder if I talked enough because maybe, just maybe, I did not talk as much as I should have. I do remember talking about it much more in the earlier years, but with time, that faded. Now that I think about it, I did not want to talk about her because deep inside, I did not want to let her go. In my mind, consciously and unconsciously, I thought that if I did not talk about her, she would be close to me and always be that way. Things changed when a wise woman during therapy persuaded me that I needed to let her go. I could only do that by going through the grief and, by talking about her, letting her out.

The thing is that losing someone we love is one of the most heartbreaking and complicated events we face. Yet, while death deprives us of a loved one's physical presence, that does not mean we have lost everything we loved about the person. With time, our relationship becomes one based on memory rather than physical presence. That being said, our loved ones may be gone, but their memories never die. Let us take a look at some ways that we can remember, honor, and always think about our lost beloveds and keep them in our memories as an integral part.

> *"Mourning never really ends. Only as time goes on, it erupts less frequently."*
>
> —Anonymous

Think about it. How do you ever find your way out of the wilderness of your grief? Several psychological models describing grief refer to "resolution," "recovery," "reestablishment," or "reorganization" as being the destination of your grief journey. These words and terms might resonate with you, and they might not, but the higher chances are that they will. You may also be coming to understand one of the most fundamental truths of grief. It is that grief never truly ends, and there is no resolution every time.

People do not just get over grief. My personal experience of losing a child tells me that a total return to normalcy after the death of someone loved is not possible; we are all forever changed by the experience of grief.

If you did not relate to the words mentioned above, you might relate to the word reconciliation, as I find it more appropriate for what occurs as you work to integrate the new reality of moving forward in life without the physical presence of the person who died. With reconciliation comes a renewed sense of energy and confidence, along with an ability to fully acknowledge the reality of death. It also creates a sense of capacity to become re-involved in the activities of living. Moreover, there is an acknowledgment that pain and grief are difficult yet necessary parts of life. There cannot be enough emphasis on the fact that grieving is the first and the biggest step into healing the scars, wounds, and voids left within and on us by the ones we loved with all our hearts.

During reconciliation, you will recognize that life is and will continue to be different without the presence of the person who died. Changing the relationship with the person who died from one of presence to one of memory and redirecting one's energy and initiative toward the future often takes longer—and involves more hard work—than most people are aware. We, as human beings, never resolve our grief but instead become reconciled to it.

We come to reconciliation in our grief journeys when the full reality of death becomes a part of us. Beyond an intellectual working through of the death, there is also an emotional and spiritual working through. What had been understood at the *head* level is now understood at the *heart* level.

In all of this, it is vital to keep in mind that reconciliation does not just happen like that. To experience reconciliation requires that you *descend*, not *transcend*. You do not get to go around or above grief – you must go through it. And, while you are going through it, you must express it enough to reconcile yourself to it. Through this, you will find that, as you achieve reconciliation, the sharp, ever-present pain of grief will give rise to a renewed sense of meaning and purpose. It is highly likely that your feeling of loss will not completely disappear, yet I can assure you they will soften. More so, the intense pangs of grief will become less frequent.

What one can do through this all is hope for continued life. This hope will emerge as you are able to make commitments to the future, realizing that the person you have given love to and received love from will never be forgotten. The unfolding of this journey is not intended to return to an old normal, rather a discovery of a new normal.

To help explore where you are in your movement toward reconciliation, the following signs that suggest healing may be helpful. You do not have to see all of these signs for healing to be taking place. Again, remember that reconciliation is an ongoing process. If you are early in the work of mourning, you may not see any signs of reconciliation. But this list will give you a way to monitor movement toward healing.

Signs of reconciliation.

As mourners embrace their grief and do the work of mourning, they can and will be able to demonstrate the majority of the following:

- A recognition of the reality and finality of the death.

- A return to stable eating and sleeping patterns.

- A renewed sense of release from the person's passing: They will have thoughts about the person, but they will not be preoccupied with these thoughts.

- The capacity to enjoy experiences in life that are normally enjoyable.

- The establishment of new and healthy relationships.

- The capacity to live a full life without feelings of guilt or lack of self-respect.

- The drive to organize and plan one's life toward the future.

- The serenity to become comfortable with the way things are rather than attempting to make things as they were.

- The versatility to welcome more change in life.

- The awareness that they have allowed themselves to fully grieve and that they have survived.

- The awareness that nobody "gets over" grief, instead they have a new reality, meaning, and purpose in their lives.

- The acquaintance of new parts of themselves that they have discovered in their grief journeys.

- The adjustment to new role changes that have resulted from the loss of the relationship.

- The acknowledgment that the pain of loss is an inherent part of life resulting from the ability to give and receive love.

Reconciliation emerges much in the way grass grows. Usually, we do not check our lawns daily to see if the grass is growing, but it does grow, and soon we come to realize it is time to mow the grass again. Likewise, we do not look at ourselves each day as mourners to see how we are healing. Yet, we do come to realize, over months and years, that we have come a long way. It is a long journey, and nobody can dictate it for us. We need to understand it is our journey, it is our grief, and the time taken to overcome it has to come on our watch. We have taken some important steps toward reconciliation.

Of course, you will take some steps backward from time to time, but that is to be expected. Keep believing in yourself. Set your intention to reconcile your grief and have hope that you can and will come to live and love again. The point I keep reiterating is that it will happen. Take your time. There are things that you can do, and there are tips and tricks that might help your cause, but at the end of the day, it is your grief, and you get to decide when it is comfortable for you to let go.

Below are some easy tips to keep their memory alive when we think of our loved one that has passed.

1. Celebrate your loved one's birthday.

Every year, take a few moments to be thankful for the life they lived and the positive ways they impacted you. You can look back on the wisdom shared, the joyful moments, the love and support you received, and you can honor those memories by sharing that wisdom, love, and support with others.

2. Host a dinner in their honor.

Choose a special day (birthday, anniversary, Mother's Day, for example) to honor your loved one's memory by inviting a group of friends to dinner. You could hold it at the person's favorite restaurant or craft a menu of dishes that your loved one particularly enjoyed, then share memories and receive support from friendships in your life.

3. Set up a permanent memorial and visit regularly.

For those who are grieving, it is often helpful to have a place to go where you feel close to the one you have lost. For many people, a memorial or a gravesite becomes that special place. If there is not a gravesite, installing a memorial bench at a significant place or planting a memorial tree may be an alternative. You could even include a memorial plaque so that anyone who passes by will be touched by your loved one's life. Also, keep in mind your loved one's preferences.

4. Create a memorial video/memory box.

This activity may be especially helpful for those with young children. Children's memories fade over time, so a memorial video or memory box can help a child hold onto memories and form a connection with the person they love and miss. The child can see his or her loved one regularly and watch the video as much as needed. With a memory box, they can touch and hold items that once belonged to the person who died and create a connection in that way.

5. Create your own tradition.

If your loved one enjoyed dominoes, play dominoes on their birthday. If your loved one enjoyed action movies, set up a monthly night to watch the newest one. Let us say your loved one enjoyed reading novels – commit to reading one a year in their memory. Did your loved one adore bananas? Set up an evening of banana-flavored foods with friends. Banana bread. Strawberry-banana smoothies. Banana pudding or pancakes. Your grandmother's banana punch. The possibilities are as unique are your loved one.

6. Visit special places.

If you and your loved one had places you always enjoyed going to together, continue to visit those places. Did you have a favorite coffee shop or bookstore? Go to those places and enjoy yourself while also setting aside time to remember your loved one. You might even consider writing them a letter each time you visit, telling them about a specific time you visited together or sharing how much you miss them.

Life goes on. Of course, you do not want to hear this right after you have lost someone, but it is also a fact that we cannot deny, neither can we sugarcoat it. The only thing we can do is that we understand that, yes, life goes on, but it does not have to go on without the thought of your loved ones. Their memories will remain embedded in and onto your heart and soul forever. We need to comprehend that death does not stop us from loving those we have lost. The love stays with us. The relationship you shared is important and worth remembering and sharing with others. We all need an outlet to express what we are feeling inside, and these activities will help you do that. By taking part in any or all of these activities, you will feel closer to your lost loved one and create forward motion in your grief journey.

Chapter 11

Her Messages

Anasofia's Soul Today

The more we dwell deeper in understanding empathy or just about being a specific kind of person, it is inevitable to talk about how generational legacy could impact the situation. Let us break this down step by step as we move through this chapter. What do you first think of when you think about generational legacy? The chances are that you think of all the traits that could possibly be passed down through our family tree. We may also think of big, blue, beautiful eyes, a good jump shot, or maybe even a natural talent for painting.

Where all of that is part of the generational legacy, it is not all that there is. Generational legacy is a thought, perspective, and belief that is emotionally or culturally passed down from our families. It is the lens through which we see the world. One that is shaped by our parents, grandparents, and key influencers. One that is influenced by culture, ethnicity, and events. We pass along through words, actions, and attitudes – consciously or not – what we know, or what we believe to be true, even if it is not.

However, it is not just the positive and influential habits or traits handed down from generation to generation. It is also all the destructive perceptual lens or relationship patterns that we are often blind to. Unfortunately, generational legacy is a gift that keeps on giving unless we can raise our self-awareness. The good news is that nobody really has to be. Even if you have experienced or exhibited destructive habits or perspectives, you do not have to continue the cycle of passing them on to your generations to come. Now that we are aware of what generational legacy is, let us take a look at its application.

We often hear from those troubled that they do not want to be like their parents in so many words: they do not want to drink as much; do not want to worry about money constantly; do not want to speak to their children the way they were spoken to. Once we dig a little deeper into what they do not like about how their parents treated them, we often find that they are navigating the world in the same way but are completely blind to it. There needs to be a better understanding of generational legacy.

To understand this better, let us look at an example to see what can go wrong. "Brittany," the mother of a four-year-old, recognizes the fact that her daughter is an anxious person. Her mother and grandmother also suffer from anxiety, so Brittany believes that anxiety is a genetic issue in her family. She feels powerless to change it, and naturally, she thinks her daughter will end up anxious as an adult due to this hereditary trait. But perhaps part of the reason the anxiety exists is that Brittany had thoughts, concerns, and fears passed down from her mother, passed down from her grandmother. Brittany has the same thought patterns her mother was raised with, and if she continues down that path of the same thoughts, her daughter will no doubt end up anxious. After all, thoughts create moods, which in turn drive behaviors.

What Brittany must do is break the generational legacy by systemically changing her thoughts. The impact of such can be exponential. Changing her core thoughts will lead to changes in her mood states (including those negative ones of anxiety and worry), her behavior, the results of her actions, and finally, her relationship with her daughter. Once Brittany achieves the self-awareness to make that change, she will recognize when her daughter begins to exhibit those same thoughts and moods and soothe her child. She can help her daughter reframe those fears and worries and guide her to think differently, therefore breaking the chain of anxiety in her family. You can take accountability to change. Even if you had a difficult childhood, this will not define the type of person you want to be and the type of life you want to live.

Most people feel that they are simply the product of their environment, history and successes and failures, and childhood; they are tethered to generational legacies and family dysfunctionality. But all of that can be overcome if you realize the problem and work to change it. It is possible to curate a new future and powerfully transform your life by reframing your thoughts and retraining your brain. You had no control over how your parents treated you, but you do have power over whether you repeat the cycle – or not.

The Link Between Parenting and Child Behavior.

Children are like sponges. They can easily pick up on good and bad behaviors and mimic what they learn at home. If a child is brought up in an environment full of tension and hostility, their future households will likely exhibit the same conflicts later in life

Research on the correlation between parenting and children's behaviors found that children who grew up with parents who were involved and authoritative repeated their parents' positive behaviors in their lives. Conversely, children with overly authoritarian or permissive parents expressed more negative behavior.

Steps To Shatter Your Legacy.

Most people are not even aware they are navigating the world through the lens of their generational legacy. But this unconscious bias hurts you, and until you become conscious of it, it is impossible to make any changes. Here are five steps you can take to stop the pattern in your family:

1. Become self-aware.

It would be best if you had the self-awareness to examine your thoughts and your perspectives. Talk to your parents and your grandparents. Learn about your ancestry. Take a hard look at your family and determine the generational legacy that is being passed along and determine where it came from. You may find that facts support the kinds of beliefs and perspectives that are passed down at one time.

"David" is worried about money. Looking at the family tree, he learned that his father was also constantly stressed about money because his grandfather lost his fortune in the Great Depression. Since his family once struggled financially, they adopted the belief that it is prudent to hoard money. That may have been the case in the past, but it is no longer true today. David is now a powerful CEO, worth millions. Even though he has plenty of money to live comfortably, he never feels like it is enough. And no matter how many more millions he makes, he will always feel like he needs more. This is an irrational fear that must first be identified through self-awareness before it can be systemically changed.

2. Take ownership of your belief systems.

Your belief systems inform how you interpret the world. You have been forming these actions, attitudes, and emotions your entire life, and they continue to be shaped today. While several factors influence your belief systems, they also influence the way you approach life.

For example, if you think you are a terrible public speaker because you flubbed a speech you gave in high school, you will likely shy away from opportunities to present your ideas to your team later in life at the office. Because you never give yourself a chance to practice your speaking skills, this perpetual fear becomes true in a vicious cycle. To assess whether your belief systems are helping or hindering you, ask yourself why you respond in the way you did in a particular situation? What thoughts were going through your brain at that time? Take responsibility for looking at the world and determining whether your generational legacy is positively serving you. If not, it is time to remove it from your belief systems, and by doing so, you are removing the barriers.

3. Travel and experience the world.

One way that generational legacies are easily broken is by exposing yourself to more of the world. Customs and traditions can be profoundly different in other parts of the world. People who travel often become more aware of and open to other customs, social norms, and ways of thinking.

4. Forgive and move forward.

Forgiveness is an important part of breaking the cycle of negative energy that can hold you back from fulfilling careers, relationships and lives. It also allows you to heal and move forward, which is important when considering family relationships.

Forgiving is not so much an act as it is a process. First, you must understand that by forgiving, you are not forgetting. You are not condoning the aggressive, offensive, or abusive behavior you have experienced. You are choosing to acknowledge and accept what happened and to move on with your life.

5. Become a model to the next generation.

Remember that wherever you have come from and whatever patterns you have learned do not hold the power to define your today or tomorrow. Your generational legacy may have been a prevalent factor for your family in the past, but it is time to start a new chapter. You have the power to create what you desire to pass down in the lives to follow, whether that is your children's or others' lives, that you impact in other ways. Being able to leave a good impact on people can be a long-term positive idea.

Our generational traits and behaviors come down to us regardless. How we want to take care of them and manage them to make us feel better and be better people is up to us. One of these big traits is being empathetic and always wanting to help people around you. The time that I spent with my daughter and the one after that was made a lot less difficult because of certain traits that people around me had. They were nicer, empathetic, and also just helpful to me in general. However, some people were neither of those things, but I guess everyone learns to live with just the best around us with time.

As this chapter concludes, the message I would give is that we must make sure that whatever shortcomings we encounter as a result of our generational legacy are not reflected upon our children. If anything at all, we must take note of all the good habits and ideas to take forward. Break the chain of toxic traits and behavior and hope to give your child the best that you can. There are ways discussed throughout the chapter in this regard and must be taken into consideration when raising children and just generally behaving around people.

Chapter 12

Letting Her Flow

Flow and Let Go

What happens between parents always impacts the children and the future that they have. It happens regardless of if the parents want it or not. This happens when you have children with special needs too. They pick up on things that you do, and it is seriously advised that one takes care of their relationship when there are children around. After Anasofia's passing, her family suffered deeply. Some days they were bitter about it. In the early years after her passing her family struggled with her memory. It was a cut deep in the flesh.

What about you? Do you struggle with memories of family relationships that feel like scars, maybe even open wounds? Are your familial bonds and losses such that they keep you wounded for as long as you can remember? These relationships as well as these losses, make and shape us, as well as those who were equally involved in the process. The fact remains that your primary relationships shape all the others.

Anasofia's parents survived her physical passing. Individually they worked and processed their feelings around grief. Sadly, they could not find a path they could share after this traumatic event, and they mutually decided to get divorced. Forgiveness, love, respect, and compassion are the words they chose for the new chapters in their lives. Dealing with Anasofia's passing and then a divorce taught me lessons that improved other relationships.

Now, how can one move towards forgiveness? Only by experiencing love and forgiveness myself could I discover how to love and forgive. My family, who shared my painful memories, helped me understand that God loved me even when I chose to reject Him. As I experienced God's forgiveness day by day, I developed a greater capacity to love and forgive others. If God chose to love and forgive me, how could I not do the same for my father?

God will always be there, offering you what is best for you. It comes down to how we accept those things from him. It all depends on how our faith directs us where we aim to be directed, and more so. How do you take hold of what God is offering you? This will sound too simple. But basically, you ask Him for it.

Christians refer to this as praying, but that means conversing with God. If you feel ready to receive the love that God wants you to experience, you could pray something like this:

Lord Jesus, I want to know you. Thank you for dying on the cross so that I could know unconditional love. I now invite you into my life and choose to hand over control to you. Make me the kind of person you want me to be.

Were you able to pray those words? If you have, you have taken a huge step of faith. God will meet you as you come to Him each day with your hopes, dreams, fears, and the pain of your past. All relationships need time and intentionality in order to grow. It is no different with God.

Everything considered, we need to know that our relationships, our traumas, and our recoveries make us the person that we are. We want to help; we want to be better versions of ourselves and do better in general. Through all of this, we need help as well. We need help from people around us. We need help from God, and most importantly, we need help from ourselves.

Being able to get over grief is not the easiest thing to do, but if we look around for assistance, there will be many hands offering help. Some of these will directly know you, while others will come your way as sheer blessings from God. You will be surprised at how much help and assistance there is, and just like that. I am hoping that this book helps you live with your special children better and also helps you understand that the loss of a child does not have to be the end of the cycle!

Chapter 13

Helping Others
is a Mission

"Being a real friend to someone who is grieving isn't easy. But I promise that if you commit to being present to someone in grief, companioning him through what might be his darkest hours, you will be rewarded with the deep satisfaction of having helped a fellow human being heal."

As we come to the conclusion of this book, I could not help but hope that this book helps you and your loved ones through the journey that you take while grieving. It is my wish to serve you on this as this book is nothing but a work of love. The love that I shared for my daughter, the love that you share with the people around you and could lose, and also the ones that you have already lost. It is love that can be your guiding light through grieving. Love for your person, love for the world around you, and love for yourself.

You see, there is incredible power unleashed when you serve someone, and that power is not just for the person that you are serving but also for yourself. Once you find yourself being in love with yourself, things tend to become easier. You grow, and you improve on yourself when you serve yourself. Serving others is synonymous with serving yourself.

Let us look deeper into this.

Over my years of grieving and loving, I have discovered that these three easy steps help every day, anywhere, to serve others in grief:

- **Listen.**

Helping begins with your ability to be an active listener. Your physical presence and desire to listen without judging are critical helping tools. Do not worry so much about what you will say. Just concentrate on listening to the words that are shared with you.

- **Have compassion.**

Give the person who is grieving permission to express their feelings without fear of criticism or judgment. Try to learn and understand. Do not instruct set expectations for and towards people to make lives difficult for them.

- **Be there.**

Your ongoing and reliable presence is the most important gift you can give. While you cannot take the pain away (nor should you try to), you can enter into it by being there for the griever. Remain available in the weeks, months, and years to come.

It is integral to understand that grieving parents tend to have an incredibly tough road ahead of them. They need all the love and support that you can give them. While you cannot make their pain go away by just being there, you can at least have your presence comfort them and make them feel safer than they would otherwise. You can be one of the brave and caring people who do not shy away from them. Trust me when I say there will be so many others who will. Offer your practical help when possible because they might need it. They might need your help with groceries, cooking, cleaning, laundry, carpooling, childcare, or other daily tasks.

You can also bear witness to their pain and understand it better. Once you understand pain better, you can help with the pain better. You can watch and listen as they express whatever they are thinking and feeling. This is not easy, but it is the kind of help that they need to begin to process their grief and move forward towards healing. In all of this, refrain from giving advice, judging, or sharing what others in their shoes have done. Instead, simply let them know they are heard and that you care.

In a similar fashion, when your spouse or partner is grieving, it is natural to want to help. Keep in mind that your job is not to take away your partner's pain, though. The hurt is natural and necessary. Instead, you can help by listening and simply being present as he encounters his pain. Be empathetic. Try to understand how your spouse is feeling from his perspective. Also, show your support in a variety of ways. Token gifts, quality time spent together, affirming words, taking care of tasks, and physical touch are all ways to show your support. If you are grieving the same loss, however, you may be so consumed by your own thoughts and feelings that you are not in a position to help your spouse. If that is the case, perhaps you and your partner can turn to other friends, a support group, or a grief counselor for help.

Let us take a look at a few more things. You can help others reach it by encouraging their deliberate mourning. They reconcile their grief by talking, writing, crying, thinking, playing, painting, or dancing it all out.

It seems obvious that acts of service help the people who are being served. When we look outside of ourselves for ways to create value for others, walk with them in times of need, and assist them in finding resources to meet their needs, most times, the people that are being helped are better off. The twist here is that, not only are those on the receiving end of the acts of service benefiting, but the person engaged in the service and the environment they are operating in are better off as well.

All of this is not just something that I am saying but something that has been scientifically tested, researched, and proven. Here are highlights of recent research studies.

- **Helping others is a contagious behavior**.

Fowler and Christakis (2010) found that when a person acts for the benefit of another person, such behavior doubles, or triples as the receiver of the benefits become givers and so on. Helping behaviors end up changing the environment in which they are conducted by creating a norm of reciprocity, whereby people feel compelled to be givers themselves.

- **When we serve others, it puts us in a good mood.**

Want to be in a good mood? Research indicates that prosocial behavior can put you in a good mood (Omoto & Snyder, 1995; Schaller & Cialdini, 1988). In one experiment, it was found that people who were allowed to help someone else reported being in a better mood than those not given the opportunity (Yinon & Landau, 1987). Another study conducted across 137 countries found that using our resources (e.g., money) to benefit others increases individual happiness (Aknin et al., 2013).

- **Giving is better than receiving.**

Focusing on others instead of yourself is more beneficial for your mental health than receiving benefits from others. After controlling for a myriad of beliefs and values, a study by Schwartz et al., 2003 found helping others related to better mental health benefits than receiving help. Research published in the *Journal of Applied Gerontology* tested the psychosomatic health of elderly volunteers who gave massages to infants and received messages themselves. Results indicated that giving massages had significantly higher physical and mental health outcomes than receiving them (Field et al., 1998).

- **Helping behaviors reduce stress.**

Numerous studies connect serving others and altruistic behavior with stress reduction (Inagaki & Orehek, 2017). A recent neuro-biological model developed by Brown and Brown (2017) suggests that caregiving behaviors likely release hormones (e.g., oxytocin and progesterone) long known to have stress-buffering qualities. Another study found that spending money on others (as opposed to yourself) was related to lower blood pressure after the action (Whillans et al., 2016).

These findings indicate the unique benefits that accrue when we serve others. It is almost as if this is a behavior we were designed to do and do regularly. Think about it. Your heart, your brain, and the science around you are all telling you the same thing.

And that my loved reader is my dream. To serve you with love every single day. Thank you Anasofia for the greatest gift. You live in my heart and many others that love you. I celebrate your life and your legacy will live on!

THE END

Acknowledgments

My family and close friends cheered me on with my idea of writing a book about Anasofia and the healing process I have gone through. Without their support, patience and love I would have spiraled down a long time ago.

My heartfelt thanks to Rodrigo. Thank you for allowing me to share the story of your daughter. Clearly, without your love, Anasofia would have never been born. I am so glad you have a beautiful family.

Thank you, Mama Paulina "Pato". Thank you for your constant overflow of love. You are my compass. Your spiritual strength, generosity, and motherly instincts always surprise me. Thank you, Papa Jorge. My sister Laura Beatriz and my brother Jorge you are the most loving siblings one could ever have. Miguel and Daniela, thank you so much for supporting them and thank you for Anasofia's cousins. Thank you to my aunts and their husbands: Laura and Roland. Marcela and Rufino. Alejandra and Salvador. Thank you, cousins, for making me laugh so much.

My life and this book could not be complete without my recent encounter with my birth father, Eduardo. I cherish every step we take in building a loving daughter-father relation.

I am especially in debt to all the Doctors, nurses, therapists, Pastors, Priests, and coaches that helped me. Rosa Julia Martinez, thank you. Lourdes Mendez, thank you.

Special thank you to my boyfriend, Darryl, for everything - and most of all for loving me and making me laugh so hard even when I am lost in translation or my many projects. The fact that you came into my life with a cadre of in-laws and extended family who laugh at my jokes and let me play horrible golf is quite a perk.

The years have passed and I am grateful for the stories many women and families have shared with me about their loss. You are too many and too numerous to be named and, in a way, you have pushed me to finalize this book. Thank you.

All of you have made my life larger and my writing and healing possible.

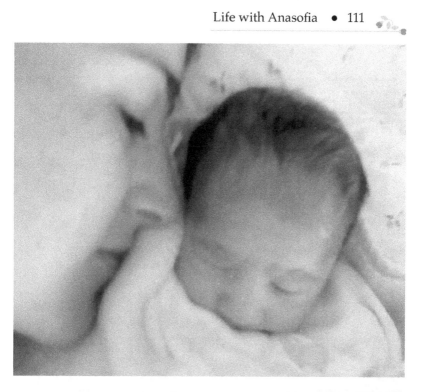

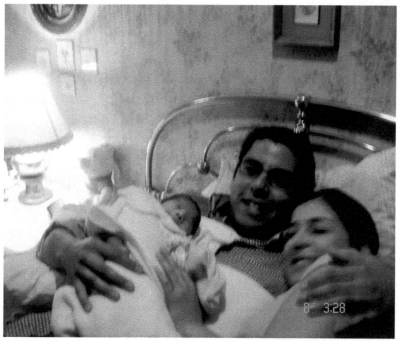

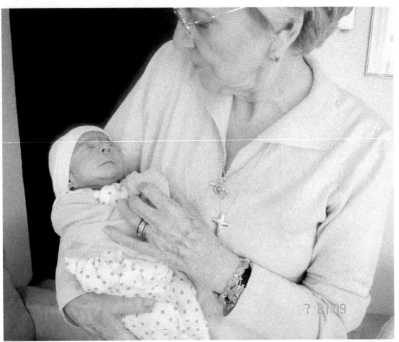

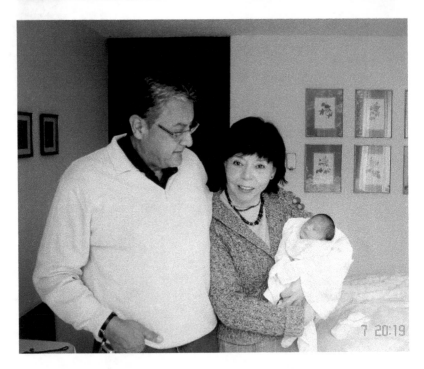

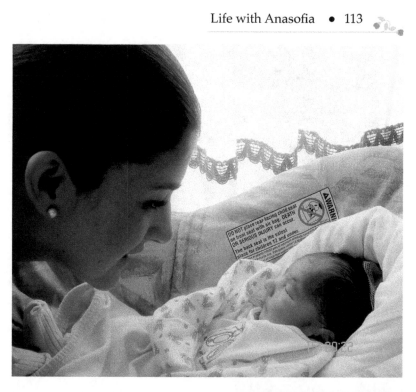

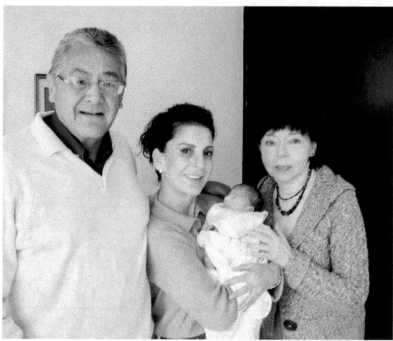

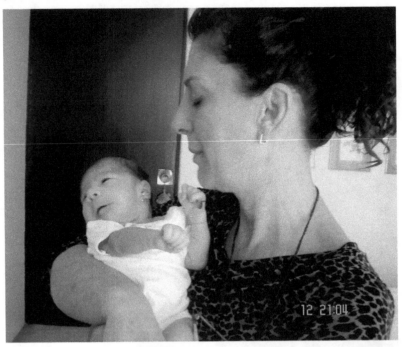

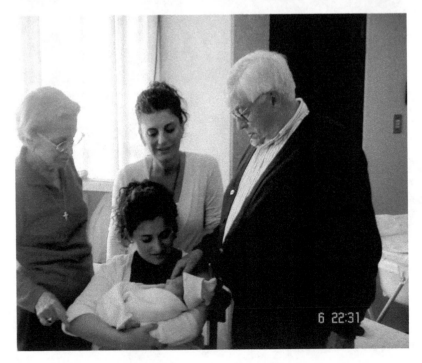

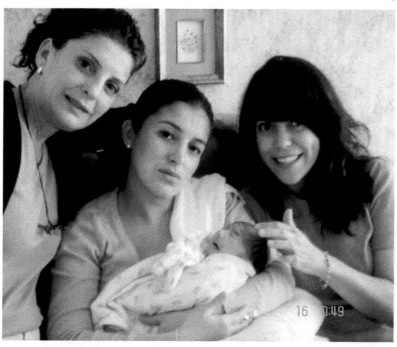

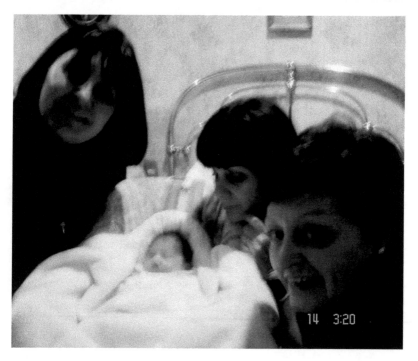

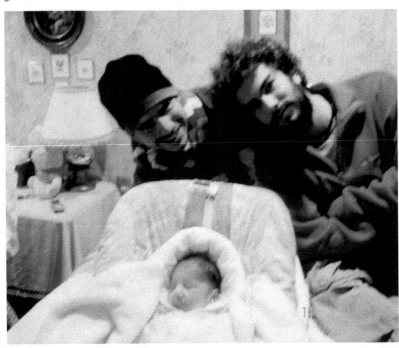

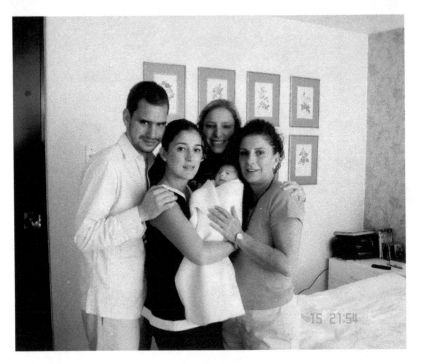

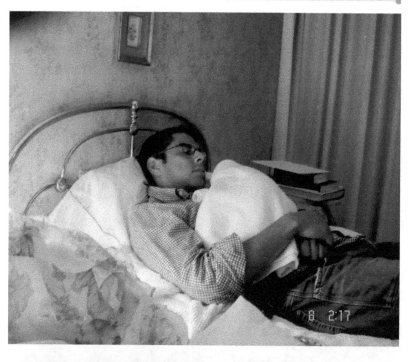

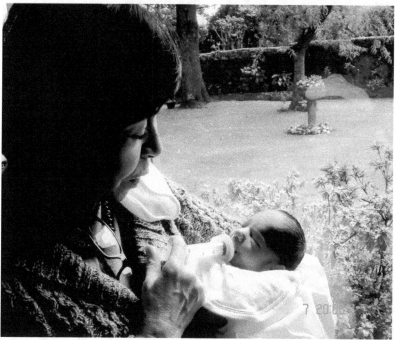

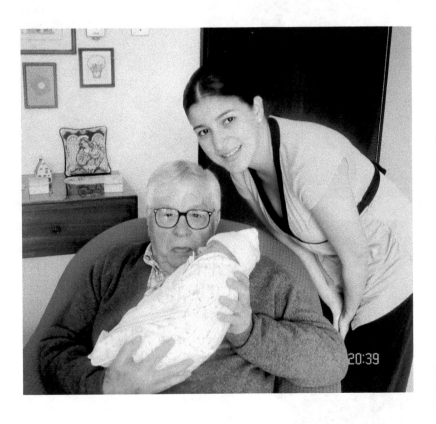